THE COMPLETE GUIDE TO INTERMITTENT FASTING FOR WOMEN OVER 50-60

Intermittent Fasting Heal Your Body for Weight Loss, Health, and Anti-Aging

Ayesha S Wakefield.

Copyright © [2024 by [Ayesha S Wakefield.)

All rights reserved. No part of this book may be reproduced or transmitted in any form or by any means, electronic or mechanical, including photocopying, recording, or by any information storage and retrieval system, without permission in writing from the author.

The exercises and information in this book are designed for healthy pregnant women who have been cleared by their healthcare provider to engage in physical activity. However, readers are advised to consult with their healthcare provider before starting any exercise program!

TABLE OF CONTENT

INTRODUCTION

I still recall the day I gave my mother the comprehensive handbook to read for women over 50–60. I was aware that this might be the answer she had been looking for because she had been having problems with her weight and general health for a long time.

I could feel her hesitancy and mistrust as we sat down to go through the guide. She had previously tried an infinite number of diets and fitness regimens, only to come away feeling discouraged and dejected. But there was something distinctive about this manual. Perhaps it was the variety of alternatives provided to fit her lifestyle and interests, or perhaps it was the way the science supporting intermittent fasting was clearly and concisely stated. Whatever it was, it seemed to work for my mom

I saw a change in her energy levels and general disposition as soon as she began putting the guide's suggestions into practice. She appeared more lively and active, as if a burden had been removed from her. Her blood sugar levels started to stabilize, and she said she felt less bloated and more focused.

But the most astounding change was still to come. My mum followed the instructions for the remaining weeks, and her body started to change. She shed some pounds, and her skin became smoother and tighter, and her hair became fuller and thicker. She felt proud and self-assured once more when individuals began remarking on how young and radiant, she appeared.

More importantly, my mother now had the skills and information necessary to manage her health. She discovered how to pay attention to her body, recognize her triggers, and adopt a more sustaining way of living. She no longer perceived herself as a victim of aging; rather, she felt in control and strong.

I can't even begin to describe my gratitude for getting to travel with my mother. It has been nothing short of miraculous to watch her develop and thrive. She has changed not only physically thanks to the entire guide to intermittent fasting for women over 50–60, but also emotionally. We now recognize and appreciate one other's accomplishments and hardships on a deeper level.

Mom, I appreciate you being receptive to our adventure. and for trusting me enough to show you the way. I am so proud of the progress you've made, and I know that this is only the beginning of an amazing new chapter in your life.

How This Book Will Help You Achieve Your Goals

giving you a thorough knowledge of intermittent fasting and its advantages, as well as useful advice and methods for incorporating it into your way of life. You can accomplish your objectives in the following ways by using this book

Sets reasonable expectations for you: Many people struggle with having lofty goals for their general health and weight loss. In this book, you'll learn how to set realistic goals and keep tabs on them.

Includes recipes and meal plans: Not knowing what to eat or how to schedule your meals is one of the major challenges people encounter when beginning an intermittent fasting routine. This book features mouthwatering and simple to prepare dishes as well as starter meal ideas.

Sets reasonable expectations for you: Many people struggle with having lofty goals for their general health and weight loss. This book gives you tips on how to set realistic goals and how to keep tabs on your development.

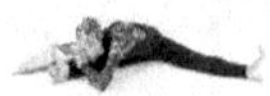

This is an image of the before and after

You'll understand intermittent fasting better after reading this book, and you'll have all the resources you need to reach your objectives. This book will assist you in reaching your goals, whether they involve weight loss, general health improvement, or just feeling more comfortable in your own skin

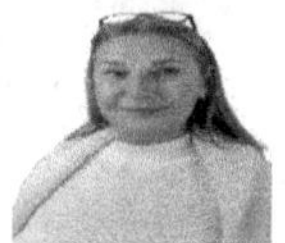

CHAPTER 1

What is Intermittent Fasting?

Simply described, intermittent fasting is a method of eating that alternates between periods of fasting and eating. Contrary to a traditional diet, which specifies what you may and cannot eat, intermittent fasting focuses on when you eat. Therefore, it instructs you when to eat rather than what or how much to eat. This strategy has been demonstrated to have various health advantages, and some people find it easier to follow than a conventional diet.

Intermittent Fasting's Health Benefits for Women Over 50-60

Due to its potential health advantages, such as weight loss, increased insulin sensitivity, and decreased inflammation, intermittent fasting (IF) has grown in popularity recently. While IF can be helpful for people of different ages, it may be especially helpful for women in their 50s and 60s. The health advantages of intermittent fasting for women between the ages of 50 and 60 will be discussed in this response, along with suggestions for how to incorporate IF into daily life.

1.**Weight loss**: Intermittent fasting has been demonstrated to aid in weight loss and may be more efficient than conventional calorie-restricted diets.

2. **Enhanced Insulin Sensitivity:** The menopause is linked to decreased insulin sensitivity, which can raise the risk of type 2 diabetes. The chance of acquiring this condition can be decreased by intermittent fasting, which has been demonstrated to increase insulin sensitivity. In obese postmenopausal women, alternate-day fasting increased insulin sensitivity, according to a research in the journal Diabetes Care.

3 **Reduced inflammation:** Chronic inflammation can cause a number of diseases, including cancer, cardiovascular disease, and arthritis, and it is a common sign of aging. The risk of these diseases can be lowered by intermittent fasting's anti-inflammatory properties. Science found that intermittent fasting reduced inflammation in middle-aged and older adults

Types of Intermittent Fasting

It's critical to select the type of intermittent fasting that is best for you as there are numerous variations on the practice. Some of the more common varieties are listed below:

- **The 16:8 Approach**: Follow a 16-hour fast followed by an 8-hour opportunity for eating.

- **The 5:2 Method:** Eat normally on the other days of the week and fast on two days each week.

- **The alternate-day** approach: abstain from food every other day.

- **The 20:4 Approach:** Follow a 20-hour fast followed by a 4-hour opportunity for eating.

Eat-Stop-Eat: Requires abstaining from food for a complete 24 hours once or twice per week, from supper one day to dinner the following.

The Warrior Diet calls for a single large meal at night within a 4-hour window of eating while undereating during the day (small portions of fresh fruits and vegetables).

* The 16/8 Method

There are various kinds. Start with the 16:8 approach. For those who are new to intermittent fasting, this is perhaps the most well-liked method and a wonderful place to start. People who are busy and don't have a lot of time to cook and prepare food should definitely consider this alternative. The 16:8 approach is simple to implement and enables you to eat three meals each day within your 8-hour timeframe. Make that you consume wholesome, balanced meals within your 8-hour interval as one thing to keep in mind.

The 5.2 diet

The 5:2 diet calls for regular eating for five days and two days of fasting with few calories. Despite initial difficulties with fasting, it is helpful for lowering blood sugar, maintaining metabolic health, and losing weight

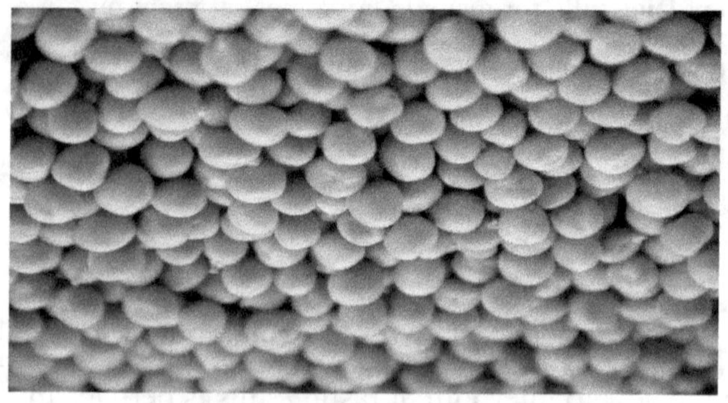

Chapter 2

Nutrition and Meal Planning

To avoid overeating and maximize the benefits of intermittent fasting, prioritize nutrient-rich foods, remain hydrated, and engage in mindful eating.

Meal Planning Strategies for Intermittent Fasting

1 **Plan Your Fasting Days:** Select the days of the week that you will fast, and then adjust your mealtimes. A 16:8 approach is one in which you fast for 16 hours and eat inside an 8-hour window. Other options include alternating days, every other day, and every other week

2. **Keep Hydrate**d: While intermittent fasting, proper hydration is crucial. Throughout the day, especially when you're fasting, be sure to drink enough water

3.. Reduce **Consumption of Processed Foods:** Processed foods typically include greater levels of harmful fats, sodium, and added sugars. Reduce your intake of these items. When possible, choose entire, unprocessed meals.

.4. **Increase Your Fiber Intake**: Fiber aids in good digestion and keeps you full. Put high-fiber foods like fruits, vegetables, whole grains, and legumes on your menu.

5. **Keep an eye on Serving Sizes:**

To maintain a calorie deficit, keep an eye on serving sizes and limit your meals. To guarantee precision, use measuring cups or a food scale.

6. **Keep It Simple:** There's no need to spend every day preparing elaborate dinners. Salads, omelets, and grilled chicken or fish can all be equally tasty and filling as more complicated dishes.

7. **Monitor Your Progress:** Regularly weigh yourself, take measures, or take progress photos to determine how well your food plan and intermittent fasting schedule are working for you.

Nutrient-rich Recipes Tailored for Women Over 50-60

Here are some nutrient-dense meals made specifically for women in their 50s and 60s, taking into account their particular dietary demands and health concerns.

Menopause-Easing Salad:

4 cups mixed greens

1 cup cherry tomatoes, halved

1/2 cup sliced red onion

1/4 cup crumbled feta cheese

1/4 cup chopped walnuts

1/4 cup chopped avocado

2 tbsp. olive oil

1 tbsp. apple cider vinegar

Salt and pepper to taste

Combine the mixed greens, cherry tomatoes, red onion slices, and feta cheese crumbles in a big bowl. Mix the olive oil, apple cider vinegar, salt, and pepper in a small bowl. Toss the salad with the dressing after pouring it over it. The flaxseeds in this salad include phytoestrogens that may help reduce menopausal symptoms. The walnuts are a fantastic source of omega-3 fatty acids, while the avocado offers beneficial fats.

Cancer-Fighting Cruciferous Vegetable Soup:

1 tablespoon olive oil

1 onion, chopped

3 cloves garlic, minced

3 cups chopped cruciferous vegetables (such as broccoli, cauliflower, kale, cabbage, brussels sprouts)

4 cups vegetable broth

1 bay leaf

1 teaspoon dried thyme

Salt and pepper to taste

Salt and pepper to taste

In a large pot, heat the olive oil over medium heat. Add the chopped onion and sauté until translucent. Add the minced garlic and sauté for another minute. Add the chopped cruciferous vegetables, vegetable broth, bay leaf, and dried thyme. Season with salt and pepper.

Smart Snacking: Healthy Choices for Fasting Days

It's critical to choose wise snacks that will give you energy and nutrition throughout fasting days or intermittent fasting without breaking your fast. For days when you're fasting, try one of these nutritious snacks:

1.1. **Nuts and seeds**: Excellent choices include almonds, walnuts, pumpkin seeds, and sunflower seeds. To keep you full, they offer protein, fiber, and good fats.

2. **Fresh fruits and vegetables** are calorie- and nutrient-efficient. To sate your cravings, munch on some carrot sticks, cucumber slices, celery, berries, or apple slices.

3.**Herbal tea:** Drink herbal teas like green tea or chamomile to hydrate yourself and help control appetite without adding any extra calories.

4. **Vegetables and hummus:** Combine your raw vegetables with a small dish of hummus for a pleasant and filling snack. Choosing nutrient-dense, satiating, and calorie-efficient foods is the key to splurging wisely on fasting days. Keep an

eye on your portion sizes and steer clear of snacks that include a lot of processed or added sugar.

intermittent fasting diet arrangement

crafting a well balance diet plan is the ultimate goal to intermittent fasting 60-50 women it's advisable to build in lean protein wholegrains, fruits, vegetables and healthy in their diet to make sure kids get enough nutrition during eating windows, meal timings and frequency should correspond with their fasting program. looking forward arraigning nutritious diet meals in forward can assist to analyze the procedure and prevent hasty food select

intermittent Fasting Recipes

Breakfast idea
Greek yogurt and berries paired with overnight oats.

spinach and avocado omelet

Almond milk, cut fruits, and chia seeds

Lunch Menu Options:

mixed greens, grilled chicken salad, and balsamic

vinaigrette

Stir-fried vegetables with quinoa

Wrap with avocado and turkey and whole-grain tortilla

Recipes for Dinner:

roasted veggies served with baked salmon

Stir-fried cauliflower rice with tofu

Marinara sauced zucchini noodles paired with lean minced turkey

Snack Ideas:

Greek yogurt sweetened with honey and almonds

Hummus paired with cucumber and carrot sticks

Almond butter on apple slices

A robust and healthful diet plan

healthy and strong meal plan

Here's an example diet plan that incorporates intermittent fasting for women in their 50s and 60s:

*Breakfast consists of Greek yogurt-topped overnight oats with sliced almonds and berries.

*Lunch consists of grilled chicken salad dressed with

cucumbers, cherry tomatoes, mixed greens, and tahini-lemon dressing

*Supper will be baked salmon over quinoa and steamed broccoli.

*Snacks: Apple with peanut butter, celery sticks with hummus, and Greek yogurt with a few walnuts. In order to supply vital nutrients and enhance general health, this diet plan places an emphasis on whole foods, lean proteins, and an abundance of fruits and vegetables.

Tips to triumph

To make the most of intermittent fasting and meal planning:

Stay Consistent: Stick to your fasting schedule and meal plan to see optimal results.

Listen to Your Body: Pay attention to hunger cues and adjust your eating habits accordingly.

Seek Guidance: Consult with a healthcare professional or registered dietitian for personalized advice and support.

Monitoring Development

It's critical to track your development in order to maintain motivation and make the required corrections. Maintain a record of your weight, energy, and general health. To guarantee long-term success, acknowledge your progress along the way and adjust your eating plan as necessary.

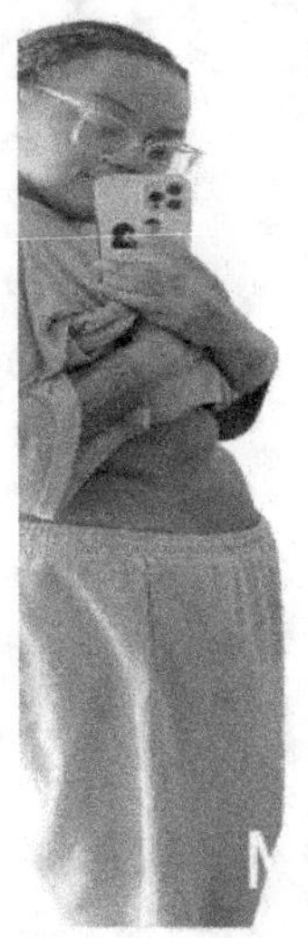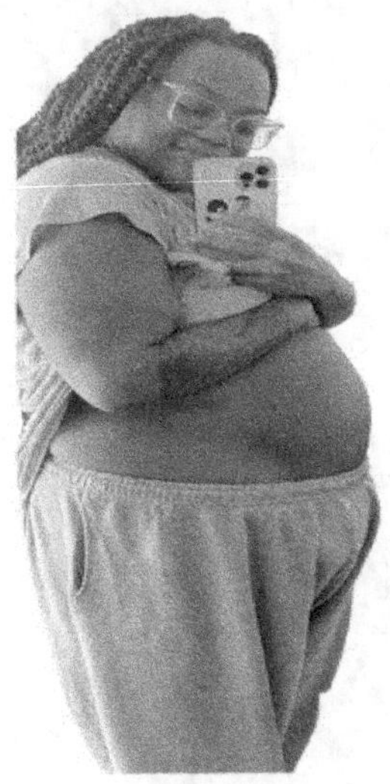

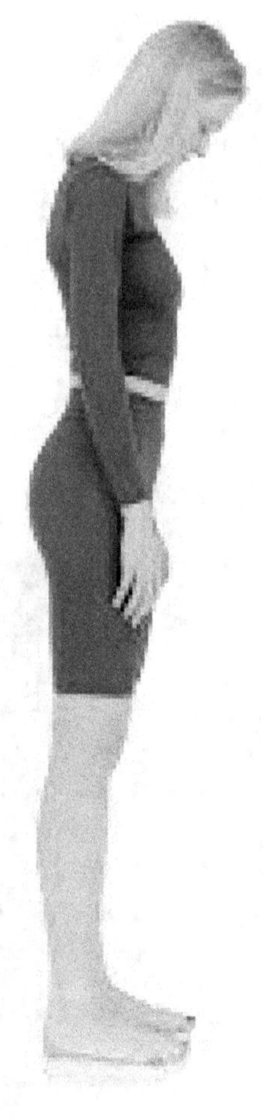

INTERMITTENT FASTING FOR WOMEN OVER 50-60

Chapter 3

Health Benefits of Intermittent Fasting

Numerous health advantages of intermittent fasting include increased metabolism, decreased inflammatory response, weight loss, improved cognitive function, and potential life extension by reducing oxidative stress and cellular aging.

*** Weight Loss and Fat Burn**

Intermittent fasting aids weight loss and fat burn by boosting metabolism, lowering insulin, curbing hunger, and activating lipolysis to break down fat for energy, making it an effective tool for weight management.

*** Improved Metabolism and Digestion**

Through adiponectin, intermittent fasting improves metabolism by controlling the breakdown of fatty acids and glucose. Additionally, it gives the digestive system a chance to recover and rest, which improves efficiency and efficacy. This is especially advantageous for people who have digestive problems.

***Hormonal Balance and Menopause**

By controlling estrogen levels, intermittent fasting helps maintain hormonal balance throughout menopause and reduces symptoms like hot flashes and night sweats. According to research, it improves sleep quality, decreases inflammatory indicators, and promotes general wellbeing and a young appearance.

*** Cognitive Function and Brain Health**

By increasing brain-derived neurotrophic factor (BDNF), which helps in the protection and repair of brain cells, intermittent fasting improves brain health. By removing damaged cells and proteins, it may lower the risk of neurodegenerative

disorders and improve cognitive function and memory.

***Snack on crisp vegetables**

like bell peppers, carrots, cucumbers, and sugar snap peas if you're eating fresh fruits and vegetables. Due to their high fiber content and low-calorie content, they can help you feel full. The natural sweetness and health advantages of fruits like apples, berries, and oranges make them excellent alternatives.

***Cottage cheese:**

Cottage cheese is high in protein and low in calories. Enjoy it on its own or with some sliced fruits for added flavor and nutrients.

Remember, the key to smart snacking on fasting days is to choose foods that are nutrient-dense, satisfying, and low in calories. Be mindful of portion sizes and avoid snacks that are high in added sugars or processed ingredients.

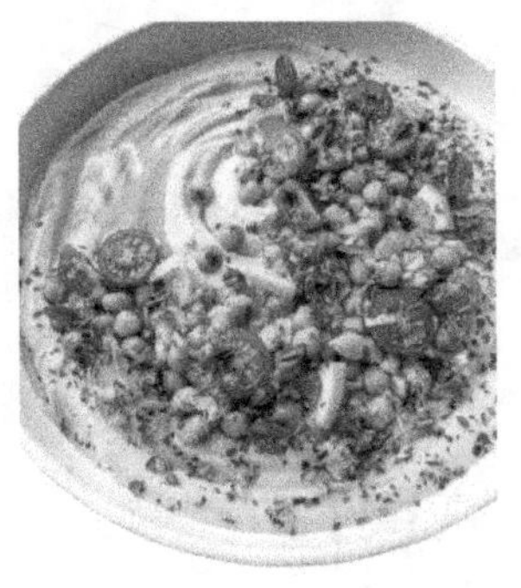

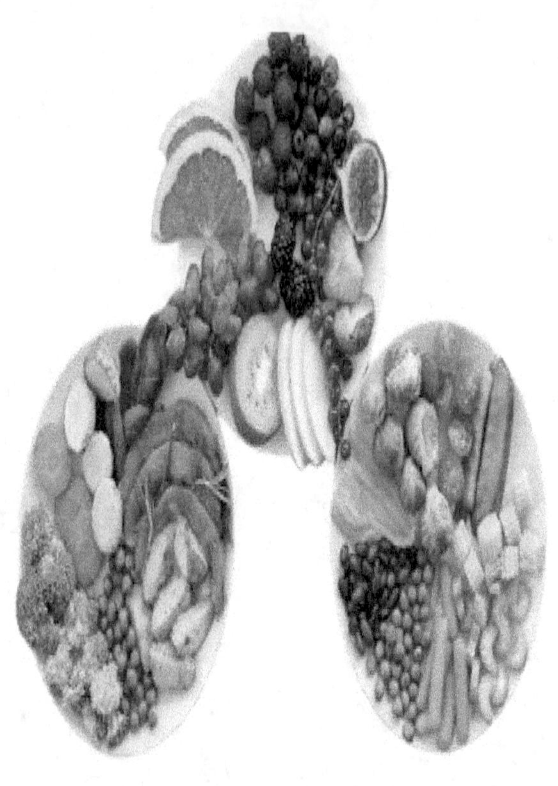

CHAPTER 4

Overcoming Challenges and Common Concerns

It's critical to recognize that intermittent fasting may be difficult at first. You might feel weak and hungry, and you might have cravings. But these signs typically go away in a few days or weeks. It's also critical to be knowledgeable about any possible hazards connected to intermittent fasting. Dehydration, low blood sugar, and electrolyte abnormalities can happen to some persons. Before beginning an intermittent fasting routine, it's crucial to speak with your doctor if you have any underlying medical concerns.

* Dealing with Social Situations and Family Gatherings

When you're trying to follow an intermittent fasting schedule, social circumstances and family gatherings can be quite difficult. It's critical to be ready for these circumstances. You might start by establishing limits and outlining your objectives for your loved ones and close friends. To have more control over what you eat, you might also want to think about bringing food to events. Finally, if the food selections don't appeal to you, don't be scared to decline. You should feel confident in your choice because it is one that is based on your health.

Troubleshooting Common Issues: A Q&A Guide

What if I am extremely hungry during fasting?

People who are unfamiliar with intermittent fasting frequently have this worry. The greatest strategy to combat hunger is to maintain a busy schedule and avoid thinking about food. You can also reduce your hunger by consuming a lot of water and herbal tea. Making sure you consume adequate calories and nutrients throughout your meal window is also crucial. Throughout your fasting window, this will lessen your hunger and keep you feeling full.

What if I get desires for unhealthful foods?

Cravings are normal and to be expected when you first begin an intermittent fasting routine, according to A. Finding healthy substitutes that will fulfill your desires is the best method to deal with them. For instance, consider eating a piece of fruit if you're desiring something sweet. Try eating almonds or roasted chickpeas if you're in the mood for something salty. Additionally, it's crucial to make sure you eat enough food during your eating window.

Another query is this:

What happens if I don't have much energy throughout my fasting window?

A: It's common to have some fatigue throughout your fasting window, especially at first. You can increase your energy levels by doing a few things, though. Try consuming a lot of water, engaging in some light exercise, and having a quick nap. Additionally, you might want to change the times of day when you eat to coincide with when you feel most energized.

CHAPTER 5

Women Over 50-60: A Guide to Intermittent Fasting and Exercise

Like with people of different ages, women over the age of 50 to 60 can benefit from intermittent fasting (IF) in a number of ways. However, it's crucial to proceed cautiously with IF and speak with a medical practitioner prior to beginning any new diet, particularly for elderly individuals. the advantage of intermittent fasting for women in this age group

***Weight control**: By limiting the amount of time spent eating, intermittent fasting helps lower total caloric intake by helping people manage their weight. women who might witness metabolic changes weight gain during and after menopause will be importantly helpful for them

***increased Insulin Sensitivity**: It has been demonstrated that IF increases insulin sensitivity. This is particularly advantageous for senior women as insulin resistance tends to rise with aging. Increased insulin sensitivity can lower the risk of type 2 diabetes and help control blood sugar levels.

***Heart Health**: According to some study, intermittent fasting may benefit heart health by lowering blood pressure, cholesterol, and inflammation. These are all critical markers for the prevention of cardiovascular

***Brain Health**: A growing body of research indicates that fasting intermittently may have neuroprotective benefits, enhance cognitive performance, and lower the risk of neurodegenerative illnesses like Alzheimer's disease.

***Length and Repair of Cells:** IF initiates autophagy, a mechanism by which cells eliminate damaged parts and mend themselves.

***Hormonal Balance**: For women going through menopause-related hormonal swings, intermittent fasting may be especially helpful in controlling hormone levels, particularly those linked to appetite (ghrelin) and satiety (leptin).

 In total intermittent fasting is strong and good for women over 50-60 it retrieve their vitality and welcome a healthier lifestyle this not about losing weight or staying fit the goal is to feel empowered strengthen and keep your head up when you welcome this intermittent fasting I know your daily eating will change but nevertheless you are building up your self-reigniting your ambition for life then you let the world know that age I s just a number. you're in charge of your health attracting your energy and be a leader for others to see and copy to all the amazing ladies out there, remember that age does not determine who you are. this intermittent fasting get use to eat welcome it because it good for your body and soul and as time goes on you will be strong illumination and unwavering resolve. Irregular fasting can help you become unstoppable throughout your greatest years, which are still ahead of you. Here's to a colorful and rewarding adventure ahead!

Creating a Schedule for Intermittent Fasting

The principles behind intermittent fasting have been established; now it is necessary to look into the nitty-gritty of making your own schedule for fasting. In this chapter, we shall discuss how to create a fast that fits your lifestyle step by step.

Define Your Objectives: Before you get ready on any fasting program, it is important to clarify what you aim to achieve. Is it weight loss, better metabolic health, more energy or increased mental sharpness? Understanding these goals will help you identify the most appropriate kind of fast as well as customize it for your personal needs.

***Choose a Fasting Protocol**: There are a number of popular intermittent fasting protocols each with its own unique twist. For example, the 16/8 method calls for 16 hours of fasting followed by an eight-hour eating window every day. The 5:2 diet allows normal eating five days out of seven and calorie restriction in two other days. On alternate-day fasting there is one day then another when a person eats normally but only drinks water throughout the whole day in between them. You might want to try different protocols until you find one that works best for you.

Determine Your Eating Window: Once you have chosen your fasting protocol, it is time to determine your eating window.tt

*Remain Hydrated**: Maintaining proper hydration during fasting times is essential for maintaining general health and wellbeing. To stave off thirst and avoid dehydration, consume lots of water, herbal tea, and other non-caloric drinks. Additionally, drinking enough of water helps reduce cravings and hunger, which makes fasting easier to control.

Plan Your Meals: After determining you're eating window, make sure your meals meet your appetite and include enough nourishment.

You will have no trouble creating an intermittent fasting plan that works for you and helps you achieve your wellness and health objectives if you just follow these guidelines and pay attention to your body's signals. We'll look at ways to get over typical obstacles and make the most of intermittent fasting in the upcoming chapter

Advanced Strategies & Methods for Becoming an Expert at Intermittent Faster

t's time to investigate more sophisticated strategies and tactics to develop your intermittent fasting practice as you gain experience with it and build a strong basis for your fasting routine. This chapter will provide techniques to help you become an expert at intermittent fasting and maximize you experience

***Try other Fasting Protocols**: While conventional intermittent fasting techniques like the 16/8 method or alternate-day fasting are beneficial, don't be scared to try other fasting protocols to see which one suits you the best. Think about implementing longer fasting windows, like 20/4- or 24-hour fasts, or investigating less restrictive methods, such time-restricted eating, which allows you to consume within a set window without necessarily fasting for long periods of time. Playing around with various fasting configurations

***Develop good eating habit** intermittent fasting makes you to have a good eating manners make you get the chance to focus on your food eating manners Take advantage of your eating window to enjoy and savor every meal, paying attention to the flavors and textures of the food as well as your body's signals of hunger and fullness. when easting don't watch or read focus on the food it bit by bit good eating habit help you to process the food faster and make you know when you are okay the important aspect of it help you to be stronger and agile

***Intermittent fasting can be used with other lifestyle** routines to maximize its effects. To enhance general health and well-being, incorporate regular physical activity, stress-management practices such as meditation or yoga, and appropriate sleep into your daily routine. These additional behaviors can improve the benefits of intermittent fasting on metabolism, energy levels, and mental clarity, resulting in a more comprehensive approach to health optimization.

Honoring Your Advancement

Respecting Your Progress for Women in Their 50s and 60s: A Handbook on Intermittent Exercise and Fasting As women grow older, they set out on a journey that is rich in knowledge, life lessons, and personal development. A critical turning point in this journey occurs between the ages of 50 and 60, at which point self-care becomes critical. This stage of life can be substantially improved by adopting practices like exercise and intermittent fasting, which foster health, energy and general wellbeing

***Self-Care significance**

Women in their 50s and 60s frequently find themselves balancing work and family obligations in addition to other responsibilities. It's critical to put self-care first in the middle of these responsibilities. Acknowledging your progress entails appreciating the importance of your health and wellness and actively caring for yourself.

*Knowing About Periodic Fasting

Because of its possible health benefits, intermittent fasting has become more and more popular in recent years. Intermittent fasting is more about when you eat than it is about what you consume. It entails alternating between eating and fasting intervals to give your body a chance to recuperate.

There are several benefits to intermittent fasting for women who are over 50–60. It could potentially lengthen life and contribute to better metabolic and cognitive wellness. Intermittent fasting may be a useful tool in your quest for optimum health if you match your eating habits with your body's natural cycles.

*Accepting Physical Activity for Health

Another essential component of a healthy lifestyle, particularly as you become older, is exercise. Frequent exercise can support the maintenance of bone density, muscular mass, and whole movement. It also contributes significantly to stress reduction, mood enhancement, and energy enhancement. A regimen that works for you and your tastes is essential for women in their 50s and 60s who want to exercise. It's crucial to maintain an active lifestyle, whether that means weight training, yoga, swimming, or walking. Exercise improves not just your physical health but also your mental and emotional wellbeing when you incorporate it into your daily routine.

***Exercise and Periodic Fasting Together**: A Powerful Combination

Combining the advantages of exercise with intermittent fasting can maximize each of them. While exercise can assist maintain lean muscle mass during fasting periods, fasting can also increase the benefits of exercise on burning fat. They foster general health and energy by working in a potent synergy.

IN TOTAL

Respecting your progress as a woman over 50–60 means accepting the path with dignity, tenacity, and self-love.

Exercise and intermittent fasting are two effective strategies that can aid you in your attempt by fostering vigor, strength, and general well-being. By adopting these habits into your daily life, you're honoring the incredible journey of women at every stage of life in addition to making an investment in your health.

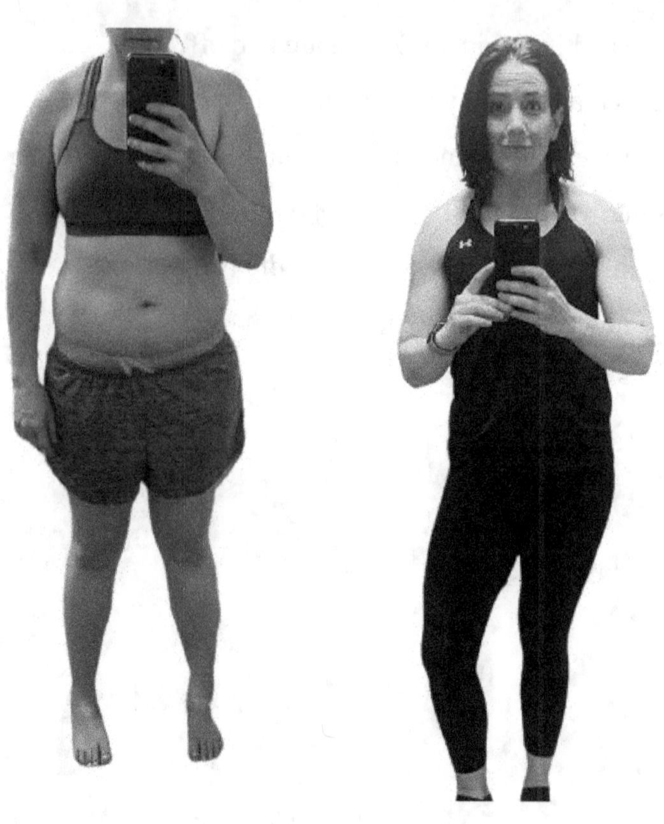

INTERMITTENT FASTING FOR WOMEN OVER 50-60

CHAPTER6

The advantage of meal planning for intermittent fasting for women over 50–60

Due to its potential for weight loss as well as its documented health benefits, intermittent fasting, or IF, has become worldwide know in this 22 century. Adopting intermittent fasting can be especially beneficial for women over the age of 50–60 since it can assist address a number of age-related health issues. But in order to get the full advantages of intermittent fasting, thoughtful meal planning must also be implemented. The emphasis of this eating logic is on timing

rather than dictating what items should be consumed. A few popular IF techniques are the 16/8 approach, which involves fasting for 16 hours and eating within an 8-hour window; the 5:2 method, which involves eating regularly for five days and reducing calories for two non-consecutive days; and alternate day fasting, which alternates between regular eating days and fasting days.

The important of Planning Meals

Although there are many health benefits to intermittent fasting, the quality of the food ingested during meal windows has a significant impact on how successful it is. This is when organizing your meals becomes essential. Women in their 50s and 60s may support their intermittent fasting objectives and make sure they're getting the nutrients they need by carefully arranging their meals. Meal planning has the following benefits

***Controlled Portions:** Preparing meals ahead of time encourages improved portion management and weight reduction by preventing overeating during eating periods.

***Nutrient-Rich Choices**: Making a plan enables you to choose foods high in nutrients, such as fruits, vegetables, lean meats, and whole grains, which promote general health And wellbeing.

***Metabolism and Satiety**: Proper meal planning guarantees a harmonious proportion of carbs, proteins, and fats—a crucial component for optimal energy, metabolism, and satiety.

***Time-saving**: Arranging meals in advance minimizes scrumptious food decisions during times of hunger and saves time.

Knowledgeable Perspective

The significance of meal preparation for women over 50-60 who practice intermittent fasting is emphasized by nutritionist Dr. Jessica Smith, who specializes in women's health:

The secret to making sure women in this age bracket follow an intermittent fasting schedule and acquire the nutrients they require is meal planning. Making balanced meals that promote bone health, hormone balance, and general well-being is made possible by it

Useful Advice for Meal Planning

When strategizing meals for intermittent fasting, keep the following in mind

Put an emphasis on entire Foods: opt for minimally processed, entire foods such fruits, vegetables, lean meats, nuts seeds and whole grains

***Incorporate Protein**: During times of fasting, meals high in protein can aid prolong feelings of fullness and maintain lean muscle mass. Add sources including fish, poultry, tofu, legumes, and Greek yogurt

Make fiber a priority. It facilitates digestion, increases feelings of fullness, and helps to maintain blood sugar levels. Consume a lot of foods high in fiber, such as fruits, vegetables, legumes, and whole grains.

Keep Yourself Hydrated: To keep hydrated and promote general health, drink lots of water throughout the day, especially during fasting.

INTERMITTENT FASTING FOR WOMEN OVER 50-60

Sample Meal Plan

Here's a sample meal plan for women over 50-60 practicing intermittent fasting:

Time   Meal

8:00 amBreakfast Greek yogurt with berries

and almonds

12:00 pm   Lunch: Grilled chicken salad with

mixed greens

vegetables, and vinaigrette

3:00 pm   Snack: Sliced apple with peanut butter

6:00 pm   Dinner: Baked salmon with quinoa and

roasted vegetables

To sum up

To sum up, meal planning is essential to ensuring that women over 50-60 years old get the most out of intermittent fasting. Reducing the risk of age-related illnesses, controlling weight, balancing hormones, and supporting health objectives may all be accomplished by women via thoughtful meal planning. Meal planning gives an all-encompassing approach to health and fitness in later life when combined with intermittent fasting.

Resolving Frequently Asked Question

When women between the ages of 50 and 60 start intermittent fasting and meal planning, they could run into a few frequent problems. Here's how to successfully deal with them

Hunger Pangs: Especially when beginning intermittent fasting, it's common to feel hungry. In between meals, stay hydrated by drinking water, herbal tea, or flavored sparkling water to help reduce hunger

*Low Energy: Feelings of exhaustion or low energy may be experienced at first when adjusting to intermittent fasting. For long-lasting energy throughout the day, make sure meals are balanced with protein, good fats, and complex carbs.

***Social Situations**: Meal planning and intermittent fasting may be difficult to follow during social gatherings and events. Make a plan in advance and bring a nutritious food to consume before or after the event.

*Honoring achievement

And lastly, it's critical to acknowledge and appreciate your accomplishments. To stay inspired and dedicated to long-term health and wellness objectives, recognize and celebrate accomplishments, whether they are related to weight reduction, energy levels, or just feeling better all over. For extra motivation and support, think about keeping track of your progress, treating yourself to non-food delights, or sharing your accomplishments with loved ones.

***Concluding Remarks of Motivation**

For women over 50–60, starting a journey of intermittent fasting and meal planning may be transforming and powerful. Women may age with energy, resilience, and grace if they adopt a proactive attitude to their health, well-being, and nutrition. Recall that self-compassion, adaptability, and constancy are the keys to success.

CONCLUSION

Last but not least, if you're a lady over 50 or 60, trying intermittent fasting can change your life. It involves a lifestyle transformation that offers several advantages, rather than only changing one's food. One thing is evident from all of the approaches and tactics we've looked at, which are customized to meet the particular requirements of women in this age range: intermittent fasting isn't only about controlling health problems or dropping pounds; it's also about regaining energy and embracing healthy living. Not only can you change when and what you eat, but you can also rewrite the story of aging by implementing intermittent fasting into your lifestyle. The concepts at play include resilience, empowerment, and accepting aging's wisdom. Hence, keep this in mind when you end this tutorial. Utilizer To live a better, happier life, keep in mind that this is just the beginning of your journey. Allow the principles of intermittent fasting to lead you to a future full of vigor, energy, and a renewed love and appreciation for life."

Despite the difficulties along the path, you have the ability to change your life in ways you never would have thought possible if you are committed to the process and persistent. Imagine having more energy than ever when you wake up in the morning, feeling energetic and full of life. Imagine yourself reaching all of your health objectives with ease, be it managing chronic diseases, losing those obstinate pounds, or just feeling better about yourself. Beyond the health advantages, though. A significant chance for personal development and self-discovery is provided by intermittent fasting. It's an empowerment journey in which you take charge of your health and pave the way for a happier, more satisfying future

Thus, keep in mind to treat yourself with kindness as you set out on this life-changing adventure. Celebrate your successes, accept the process, and take lessons from failures. Above all, have faith in your capacity to succeed in spite of whatever challenges you may encounter. Ultimately, The Complete Guide to Intermittent Fasting for Women Over 50–60 is a road map to a better, happier you, not simply a book. Take the first step now and start the trip today,

Testimonials and Success Stories

It can be quite exciting and motivating to read about other people's experiences with intermittent fasting. It can provide you inspiration for how to make your personal intermittent fasting plan successful and make you feel like you're not alone on your path. You can also see the many advantages people have encountered, such as weight loss, more vitality, and greater mental clarity.

An example of a buddy who successfully used intermittent fasting is given here:

I'm so glad I gave intermittent fasting a try despite my initial skepticism. I first tried the 16:8 approach, which required me too fast for 16 hours before eating for 8 of those hours. It didn't take me long to see a difference. I felt less hungry at night and had more energy and concentration during the day. My weight and general health started to change after a few weeks. I'm really happy I gave intermittent fasting a shot because I feel fantastic!

I also want to share with you a reference from a relative.

Intermittent fasting has changed my life in ways that I never would have imagined. It took some getting used to not eating for extended periods of time, but as I established a schedule, it was lot simpler. I've shed a large amount of weight, and I also have more energy and am not as hungry all the time. I feel in charge of my life and health more than anything else, though. I'm very appreciative that you gave me the chance to try intermittent fasting because I'll never go back!

I have many testimonies but I just decided to share a few of them without contradiction it really works and you will see the result in no time thanks for reading and applying

HAPPY READING

www.ingramcontent.com/pod-product-compliance
Lightning Source LLC
Chambersburg PA
CBHW051707250726

48653CB00007B/2894